THE
ALEXANDER
TECHNIQUE

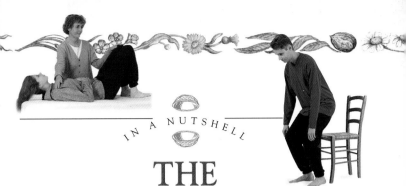

IN A NUTSHELL

THE
ALEXANDER
TECHNIQUE

A STEP-BY-STEP
GUIDE

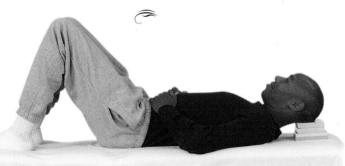

AILSA MASTERTON

ELEMENT

SHAFTESBURY, DORSET • BOSTON, MASSACHUSETTS • MELBOURNE, VICTORIA

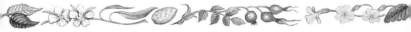

© Element Books Limited 1998
First published in
Great Britain in 1998 by
ELEMENT BOOKS
LIMITED Shaftesbury,
Dorset, SP7 9BP

Published in the USA in 1998 by
ELEMENT BOOKS INC
160 North Washington Street,
Boston, MA 02114

Published in Australia in 1998 by
ELEMENT BOOKS LIMITED
and distributed by Penguin Australia Ltd
487 Maroondah Highway, Ringwood,
Victoria 3134

Designed and created with
The Bridgewater Book Company Ltd

ELEMENT BOOKS LIMITED
Editorial Director Julia McCutchen
Managing Editor Caro Ness
Production Director Roger Lane
Production Sarah Golden
Project Editor Katie Worrall

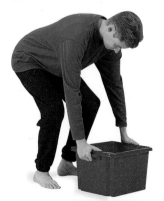

THE BRIDGEWATER BOOK
COMPANY LTD
Art Director Terry Jeavons
Designer Glyn Bridgewater
Page layout Glyn Bridgewater
Managing Editor Anne Townley
Project Manager Fiona Corbridge
Picture Research Lynda Marshall
Three-dimensional models
Mark Jamieson
Photography Ian Parsons
Illustrations Andrew Kulman
Printed in Great Britain by
Butler & Tanner Ltd, Frome
British Library Cataloguing in
Publication data available

Library of Congress Cataloging
in Publication data available

ISBN 1-86204-195-4

The publishers wish to
thank the following for the
use of pictures: Hutchison:
23; Zefa: 7TR,
7B,16TL, 28B.

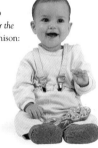

Special thanks to:
Ailsa Masterton,
Lily Adams,
Maria Anderson,
Paul Castle,
Robert Chappell,
Jonathan Dean, Jane Hallwood,
Julia Holden, Natalie Jerome, Darren Law,
Rebecca McGratty, Claire Morgan,
Peggy Painter, Neil Redfern, Mat Rose,
Jacob Swirsky, Art Terry, Sammy Thomas
for help with photography.

Crescent Clinic, Brighton, UK
and Robert Harding, Brighton, UK
for help with properties.

Contents

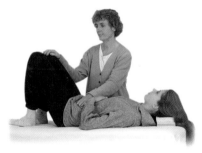

What is the Alexander Technique?

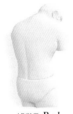

ABOVE: **Back problems are common, with up to 60 per cent of adults suffering from them.**

"EVERY MAN, *woman and child holds the possibility of physical perfection; it rests with each of us to attain it by personal understanding and effort.*"

FREDERICK MATTHIAS ALEXANDER

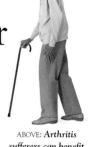

ABOVE: **Arthritis sufferers can benefit from practising the Alexander Technique.**

Most of us, when we are undertaking simple tasks, physical or mental, do so with undue levels of tension which limit our performance. The result may be a stiff neck, round shoulders, poor posture, lower back pain, or other problems that hamper us in some way. The Alexander Technique gives us the choice to change this – to change the way in which we hold ourselves, walk, sit, stand, or operate at work, so that movement becomes freer and we begin to regain our natural poise and balance. Through a gradual process of re-education we can become more self-aware, learn to recognize harmful habits we may have developed over many years, and work toward changing our approach.

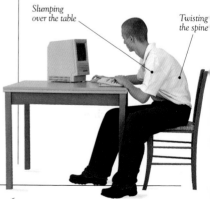

Slumping over the table

Twisting the spine

RIGHT: **It is easy to fall into bad habits at home, at school, or at work.**

Over the last decade many people have become increasingly aware that mental, physical, and spiritual health are all connected. Alexander teachers work with the whole person, linking the way in which our thought processes, emotions, and feelings affect our bodies.

The Alexander Technique is taught on a one-to-one basis. Lessons focus on improving physical and mental well-being by reducing muscular tension and working with the relationship between the head, neck, and back.

WHO CAN IT HELP?

People who may benefit from the Alexander Technique generally fall into three categories.

☞ Those who suffer from back pain, neck and shoulder tension, stiffness in the joints, poor posture, breathing problems, and arthritis.

☞ Those who have problems generated by the work they do, such as poor posture or repetitive strain injury. Dentists, carpenters, computer operators, builders, actors, singers, dancers, musicians, and sportspeople, who rely heavily on their bodies functioning well, all benefit from the Technique.

☞ Those who may not have identified a particular problem but have heard about the benefits of the Alexander Technique. Our holistic age has made people aware of the need to "take care" of themselves rather than wait until problems occur, and teachers increasingly find that this is the reason people seek their help.

ABOVE: *Dancers need to maintain peak physical fitness. The Technique helps to achieve this.*

RIGHT: *For sportspeople, working with the technique can enhance performance and prevent injuries.*

THE ALEXANDER TECHNIQUE WILL HELP YOU TO

☞ become aware of yourself as a whole – your mind, body, and spirit.
☞ prevent undue strain and tension in your body.
☞ become aware of how you approach daily activities.
☞ change persistent harmful habits.

A short history

ABOVE: *Frederick Alexander (1869-1955). The Technique sprang from problems with his voice and throat.*

THE ALEXANDER TECHNIQUE *was developed by Frederick Matthias Alexander, an Australian actor and reciter, who was born in 1869. By inspired observation he discovered that the way in which the head was balanced upon the top of the spine, and the relationship between the head, neck, and back, had a profound effect on the efficient functioning of the whole person.*

In the early days of his acting career Alexander started to experience periods of hoarseness during his performances. His physicians diagnosed inflamed vocal cords and prescribed various treatments and rest, but his condition grew worse and the medical experts could not offer a long-term solution. Alexander concluded that something he was doing in using his voice was the cause of the trouble, and he resolved to find the root of the problem himself.

Alexander's problems were not initially obvious during ordinary speech, but through the use of mirrors, he observed a distinct pattern when he was reciting. He discovered that he

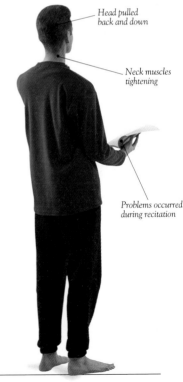

Head pulled back and down

Neck muscles tightening

Problems occurred during recitation

pulled back his head, depressed his larynx, and sucked in air through the mouth producing a gasping sound. He went on to observe that in pulling back his head he tightened his neck muscles, bringing his head back and down on to his neck, which made him shorter in stature.

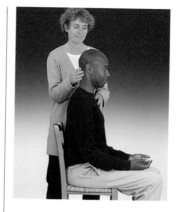

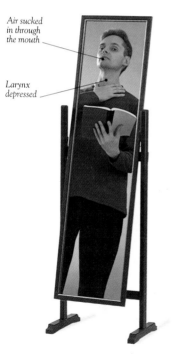

Air sucked in through the mouth

Larynx depressed

ABOVE: *Recreating Alexander's discovery of the cause of his inflamed vocal cords.*

Over many years of careful self-observation, he developed an understanding of the way in which the mind and body work together, and in particular the relationship between the head and neck, and its effect on the functioning of the rest of the body. From this he formed the basis on which the Alexander Technique is taught. In 1904 he moved to England, where many prominent people of the time showed a great interest in his work. In 1932 he started a school to train teachers and continued to develop the Technique until his death in 1955.

ABOVE: *Alexander teachers work together with their pupils, showing them how to think consciously about themselves.*

Alexander's discovery

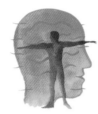

ABOVE: *The Alexander Technique views the mind and body as inextricably linked.*

THE ALEXANDER TECHNIQUE *works on the principle that the mind and body form one complete and integrated whole. Today, with the advances in psychosomatic medicine and the development of body-oriented therapies, this principle does not seem so radical, but when Alexander was writing at the turn of the century, his holistic theories were considered revolutionary.*

Alexander discovered that most people, to a greater or lesser degree, retract their head, and that this becomes even more evident when they make a movement. He wrote: "If you ask someone to sit down, you will observe, if you watch their actions closely, that there is an alteration in the position of the head, which is thrown back, whilst the neck is stiffened and shortened." This in turn puts pressure on the rest of the spine, causing distortion in its natural tensile quality, and has an effect on the rest of the body – there is

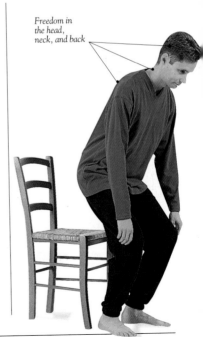

Freedom in the head, neck, and back

RIGHT: *Maintaining poise and balance whilst going into movement. (See also the section on sitting, page 47.)*

THE HEAD, NECK, AND SPINE

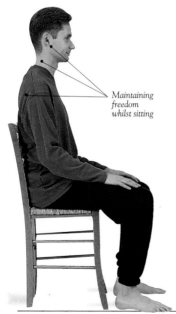

Head is balanced freely on top of the spine

Head is pulled back, exerting pressure on spinal column

Spine is able to function well

ABOVE: **Anatomical differences between the head going forward and up, and being pulled back and down.**

Maintaining freedom whilst sitting

less space for the internal organs to operate, the lungs are restricted, and the limbs are affected. When this pattern develops in the body, natural poise and balance are lost, and a variety of problems develop.

THE WHOLE PERSON

If we think of ourselves as an integrated whole, we are not just looking at the body, but at the thoughts and emotions that make us the people we are. Alexander talked about the "self" to describe this wholeness.

The way we move when engaged in physical activity is influenced by our mood: we are talking about all that goes into influencing movement – the energy it takes for us to move. When working on himself in the initial stages, Alexander found that if he consciously tried to put his head in a different position he still created muscular tension, but if he "thought" about releasing the tension in his neck muscles, his head naturally went forward and up. If he then extended the thought process to the rest of his body, the tension overall was reduced.

USE AND MISUSE

Alexander talked about "use" to describe this process of consciously thinking about approaching activity: "When I employ such phrases as, 'I directed the use,' I wish to indicate the process involved in projecting messages from the brain to the mechanisms, and in conducting the energy necessary to the use of these mechanisms."

For the most part we pay little attention to our approach when performing activities. We may remember to be careful when lifting heavy objects, or think about how we might approach a particular movement in a game of sport, but often we give it little thought.

Alexander described this lack of thought as "misuse," and recognized that only by bringing our approach into consciousness could we make changes. He noted: "I had to admit that I had never thought out how I directed the use of myself, but that I used myself habitually in the way that felt natural to me."

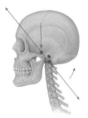

RIGHT: *When the head is balanced and the neck muscles released, the head is going forward and up.*

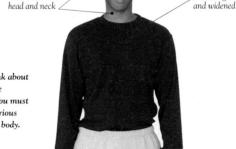

Freedom in the head and neck

Back lengthened and widened

RIGHT: *Think about how you are standing. You must consider various parts of the body.*

BREAKING BAD HABITS

Alexander found that habits were difficult to break. He had worked out that in order to make changes he needed to do things differently, but found that despite trying to do this, he failed. He realized that before making changes he had to inhibit his old pattern, give directions for the neck to be free, the head to go forward and up, and the back to lengthen and widen, which then resulted in a freer head–neck balance.

In his approach to change, Alexander also discovered that "feelings" are unreliable. We depend upon our feelings to inform us about how we are doing things – if it feels right it must be right – but it is through the force of our habits that we reach this conclusion. For the most part, we are totally unaware of habits that have developed, or that they may be unhelpful. If a person has developed the habit of raising one shoulder higher than the other, they are quite likely to be unaware of it, and for them it feels normal. When a teacher points this out and allows the shoulder to come back into balance, the pupil will initially experience this as being out of balance.

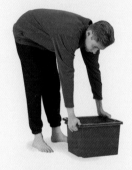

THINKING OUT YOUR APPROACH

ABOVE: *The wrong way to pick something up: lifting with undue strain and tension.*

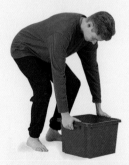

ABOVE: *The right way to do it: maintaining co-ordination of the head, neck, and back while lifting.*

DEVELOPING HABITS

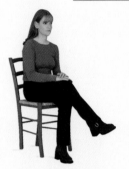

ABOVE: *Sitting with legs crossed at the knee.*

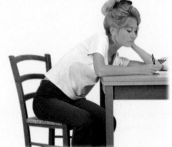

ABOVE: *Slumping over a desk, and twisting the spine.*

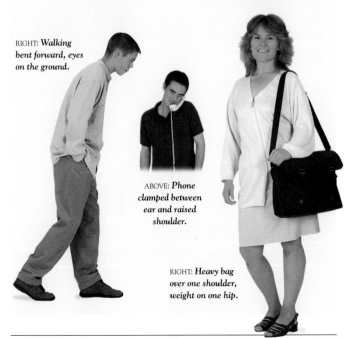

RIGHT: *Walking bent forward, eyes on the ground.*

ABOVE: *Phone clamped between ear and raised shoulder.*

RIGHT: *Heavy bag over one shoulder, weight on one hip.*

CHANGING OUR APPROACH

So how did Alexander's discoveries translate into what is today taught as the Alexander Technique? The key points are:

☞ Our approach to most activity is habitual and unconscious.

☞ The relationship between the head, neck, and back is of vital importance.

☞ The head and neck joint affects the whole person.

☞ Our thoughts, feelings, and emotions affect the level of tension in the body.

☞ We can consciously change our habitual approach to activities.

☞ By giving ourselves "directions" (projecting messages from the brain) we can change the way we "use" ourselves.

☞ We need to stop and think about how we are going to approach any movement or activity before starting it.

It is impossible to make these changes on our own – we need to work with an Alexander Technique teacher to guide us through the process.

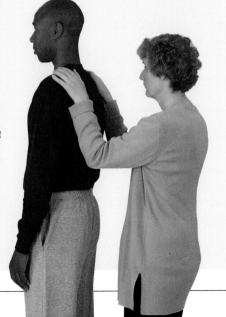

RIGHT: *An Alexander Technique teacher will work with you on your habitual responses.*

Why do we need the Alexander Technique?

ABOVE: *The modern environment generates stresses, both physical and mental.*

THE LIFE WE LEAD TODAY *is stressful and demanding, and we have to cope with constant changes as society evolves and develops. Our activities now are a far cry from the times when we lived in a more natural environment, constantly on the move hunting for food.*

As a species, we changed from hunter-gatherers to farmers over a very short period of time. Then came the Industrial Revolution, the technological revolution, and now we have moved further and further away from daily physical activity in order to survive. As Alexander observed: "Man has been and still is unable to adapt himself quickly enough to the increasingly rapid changes involved in that plan of life which we call civilization."

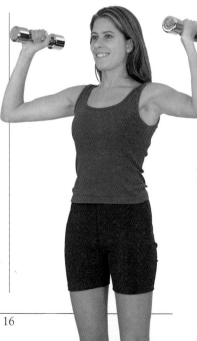

RIGHT: *Some modern forms of exercise put too much strain on certain parts of the body.*

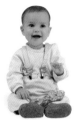

RIGHT: *A baby is able to maintain a poised head through balance rather than muscle tension.*

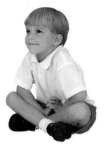

RIGHT: *At school, children often sit on the floor to listen to stories. This encourages slumping and hunched shoulders.*

CHILDHOOD

As young children we have grace and freedom of movement: bending, squatting, reaching, sitting with little effort. Watch small toddlers move with ease, sit on the floor in an upright position with no problem, squat to reach a toy, and constantly move with absolute freedom as their curiosity helps them to discover this world they inhabit.

By the time children reach school, even in the first year, they already find it difficult to sit on the floor without slumping, many have started to develop round shoulders, and others are starting to hunch the shoulders upward toward their ears. With the onset of puberty other problems follow

ABOVE: *Toddlers maintain an upright position with ease and freedom.*

and the teenage slouch is developed, resulting in twists in the spine and tension in the neck. Many young people experience tremendous growing spurts in a short space of time and find it difficult to know quite what to do with this new body, so they will often try to minimize it by sinking down, pulling in the shoulders, and slumping into chairs.

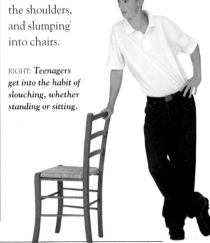

RIGHT: *Teenagers get into the habit of slouching, whether standing or sitting.*

LIFESTYLE

We now lead very sedentary lives, bent first over tables at school, then over office desks, computers, shop counters and production lines. We use our minds more than our bodies for most of the day, thus encouraging the separation of mind and the body. We have cars, supermarkets, telephones, new technology – many conveniences which allow us to expend very little physical energy in order to go about our daily activities.

This modern lifestyle takes its toll on our mental, physical, and emotional health, and as a result we develop undesirable habits which limit our potential.

WHY OUR BODIES CHANGE

- We sit at tables at school for many hours each day.
- In our working life, we spend a large proportion of our time sitting at desks, driving cars or sitting on trains.
- We are often in a constant state of stress.
- Our relaxation time involves little or no physical activity.

STRESS ON THE BODY FROM A SEDENTARY LIFESTYLE

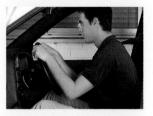

ABOVE: *When driving, we lean forward over the wheel, and tense our neck and shoulders.*

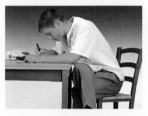

ABOVE: *We often sit badly while working at a desk, hunching over and twisting the spine.*

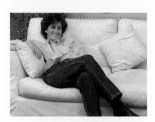

ABOVE: *We may think we are relaxing, but the spine is under stress when slouched in an easy chair.*

STRESS

Stress is also a unique feature of our life, and it is very different from the stress experienced by our forebears. In the early days of mankind, the stress of finding food and surviving was matched by the enormous physical demands on the body – which counter-balanced the stress. Today we live in noisy, hectic environments, with enormously demanding tasks and deadlines, and an overload of information. When faced with a stressful situation, adrenaline is released from the brain, which in turn releases extra blood to the muscles and increases the heartbeat. If there is no release from the stress, harmful effects build up in our bodies.

At the end of the day we tend to settle in front of the television, or sit down for a meal or a drink. Adrenaline levels remain high and our muscles can stay in a heightened state of tension. Many of us have lost the ability to let go of mental, physical, and emotional tensions.

FIGHTING BACK

The Alexander Technique helps us to counteract the adverse effects of modern life and work on the relationship between what we do and how we do it. The approach to many of our physical activities is unconscious and can become harmful over time. With the Technique we learn how to let go of long-held tensions, both mental and physical, and allow ourselves to experience a greater ease and freedom in our movements.

LEFT: *At the end of a hard day, the effects of stress on the body will manifest themselves in aches and pains.*

Who is it for?

THE ALEXANDER TECHNIQUE *is suitable for almost anyone, of any age, and increasingly people are coming to it for its general beneficial effects. As we learn to take responsibility for our own health, and to understand our bodies, the need for preventive medicine has become obvious.*

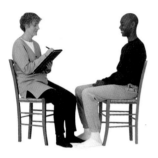

ABOVE: *Alexander teacher and pupil at the first consultation. Find a qualified teacher through the national association.*

People come to the Technique with a wide range of health problems, from back pain, shoulder tension, posture trouble, stiff joints, and breathing difficulties to general stress. The teacher's approach is not to offer an instant cure or even to focus on the problem itself, but to consider what is happening – what is the pupil doing to cause the problem? The teacher examines the problem in a wider context.

RE-EDUCATION

An Alexander teacher will work with pupils individually to help them understand how they are "misusing" themselves. However, pupils also need to take responsibility for themselves. Pupils who observe the way they "use" themselves, stop and think about how they are doing something, and think about how they could do it differently, are likely to make more progress. This is why the Technique is considered a process of education and not a therapy.

Traditionally, actors, singers, sportspeople, dancers, and musicians have practised the Technique, and it is part of the syllabus in many colleges of music and drama. Today, anyone who relies on their body to perform well, in order to make a living, to look after children, or to enjoy life to the fullest, can become involved.

WIDER EFFECTS

Around 60 million working days are lost each year through back pain, and that figure is rising. Those lost days cost the economy around $5.2 billion (£3 billion). On its own, that amount is shocking, but think of the days lost through related illness. How much money is being lost through lack of effective diagnosis and treatment for back pain? The US National Center for Health Statistics reports that back pain is the sixth most common reason for visits to the emergency room, and accounts for 13 million visits to general physicians' offices each year.

By learning the Alexander Technique most people are able to return to work, and many chronic (long-term) sufferers of back pain and joint problems experience few or no symptoms again. People with breathing difficulties learn to manage them, and highly stressed people are able to reduce their stress. When difficult situations arise, they are able to stop and deal with them with a greater sense of calm. For most people receiving lessons there is a feeling of being energized, a sense of calm, a greater feeling of well-being, and an ability to cope with life a little better.

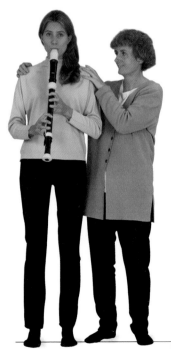

LEFT: *Alexander teachers can give advice about improving the way you hold yourself for many activities.*

The mind~body relationship

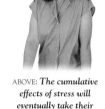

AT THE BEGINNING of his process of discovery Alexander said: "I... believed that human ills, difficulties and shortcomings should be... dealt with on specifically 'mental' or 'physical' lines." But he later found "that it is impossible to separate 'mental' and 'physical' processes in any form of human activity."

ABOVE: *The cumulative effects of stress will eventually take their toll on mind and body.*

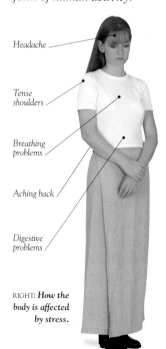

Headache

Tense shoulders

Breathing problems

Aching back

Digestive problems

RIGHT: *How the body is affected by stress.*

A HOLISTIC VIEW

Most people know very little about the body and how it works – they take it to the doctor when it goes wrong, in the same way they might take the car to the garage. They know they get aches and pains, that they might be tense at times, they might even exercise, but they make no connection with the mind, or think that they can exert any control over the body.

When people work in stressful conditions they react in a variety of ways, at times dealing with the situation really well, but often finding that the demands made upon them have exceeded their ability to cope. It is when this happens that they feel stressed, and it is this feeling of being overwhelmed that will then start to affect the body. Responses vary, but they may experience tense shoulders, headaches, a stiff neck, an aching back, digestive problems. They know that the overwhelming demands being made upon them affect the body, but rarely make the connection between the body, their attitude, and mental state.

THOUGHT AND ACTION

Alexander teachers bring together the mind–body connection. They use their hands in gently guiding the body and giving verbal explanations and directions to their pupils, who then learn how to combine their thoughts with activity. In this way, thought processes and the functions of the body work in harmony and become an integrated whole.

THE MIND–BODY RELATIONSHIP

In many cultures the mind–body relationship is an intrinsic theme, and is often part of a daily ritual. But in Western society, a tremendous division has been forged between the mind and the body, and this is exacerbated by the preoccupation with new technology, computers, television, and shopping as major recreational activities, and the decline in physical activity. Many people are seeking ways to redress the balance, through alternative therapies such as the Alexander Technique, meditation, dance, and various forms of body work.

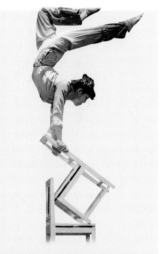

ABOVE: *The poise and suppleness of a Chinese acrobat. Eastern cultures have traditionally been more able to balance mind and body.*

How does the Technique help?

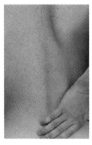

ABOVE: *Backache is an obvious candidate for the Alexander Technique: it can be dramatically reduced after several lessons.*

PEOPLE COME TO THE *Alexander Technique* for many reasons, with a variety of problems, and often through a circuitous route. But all of them come because they know there is something wrong with their body – they find it is not working in the way they would like it to.

For some people the change after lessons can be dramatic – a frozen shoulder is eased, acute back pain is reduced, headaches subside, stress becomes manageable, stiff necks are released. Others notice changes in their mental and emotional states – they get less agitated, they become more relaxed, they slow down. Sometimes the changes are more subtle and gradual, and can contribute toward life changes.

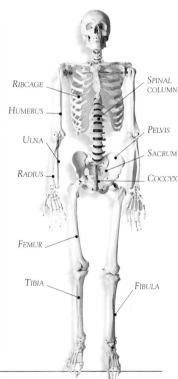

RIBCAGE

SPINAL COLUMN

HUMERUS

ULNA

PELVIS

RADIUS

SACRUM

COCCYX

FEMUR

TIBIA

FIBULA

RIGHT: *To understand the Technique a working knowledge of the skeleton is vital.*

SOPHIE'S STORY

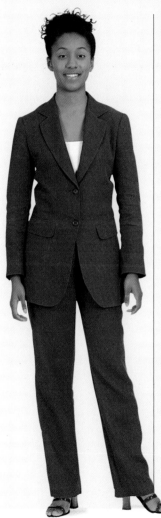

Sophie was in her early twenties. She had experienced difficulties with breathing when taking voice lessons some years ago, and her singing teacher had recommended the Alexander Technique. She wanted to start singing again and realized she needed to work with her breathing. Sophie was quite tall. She had pulled her shoulders in so much that she had developed a pronounced hump in the upper back, and her neck was fixed and tense, all of which restricted her breathing. She also had long slender toes, which were gripping so tightly that they no longer lay flat and were fixed at the middle joints.

We worked together for a year, until she moved abroad, during which time her shoulders opened out and the curvature disappeared. At this point she had to buy new clothes to fit her "new" body. Her toes gradually unfurled, although not completely, her breathing improved, and she gave up smoking. Not only were there physical changes, but she decided to go to a counselor and became more confident, clearer about who she was and less fearful. She decided to leave a fairly boring job and go back to college.

LEFT: *After treatment, Sophie was able to shrug off her former problems.*

DAVID'S STORY

When David came for lèssons he was in a lot of pain and had literally not sat down for six months. He had stopped working and was only able to kneel or to lie down. His X-ray showed two pear-shaped discs in the lower back. He had been working with an exercise routine based on the Pilates Technique and had also been to an osteopath, and although some of it helped he was still unable to sit. His pain was such that he had become fearful about even attempting to sit, so the first lesson was spent standing and lying down on the table. However, during his third lesson, working very gently and slowly bending at the hip joint, he surprised himself by actually sitting in the chair. His major goal had been to drive again, about which he was cautious, worried that he might undo the good work. Within three months he was driving again and leading a fairly normal life.

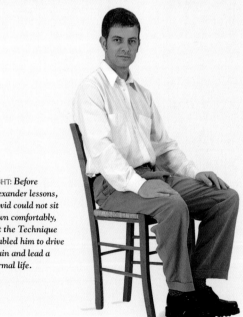

RIGHT: *Before Alexander lessons, David could not sit down comfortably, but the Technique enabled him to drive again and lead a normal life.*

ROSA'S STORY

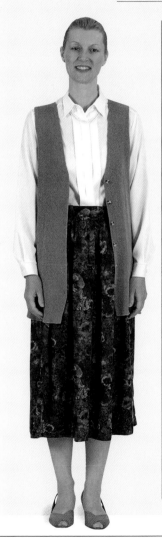

Rosa was the head teacher in a busy elementary school and had been off work for six months. A friend had given her two books on the Alexander Technique to read, and she had come to an introductory talk on the Technique, at which point she had decided with some cynicism to try lessons. She had two slipped discs in the lower spine and had spent a large proportion of the six months off work lying down. She found sitting very difficult and painful. She was unable to drive, walked extremely slowly, and preferred to take taxis rather than buses to avoid being jolted too much.

She started coming for two lessons a week and within two months decided to return to work. Her problems were not yet solved, but she felt she could work and with careful thought "manage" her back. We worked together for just over a year, at which point she decided to take early retirement. She still treats her back with great respect, but is able to lead a full and active life, swimming daily, working in her garden, and taking long country walks.

LEFT: *Rosa used the Technique to actively "manage" her back whilst working toward recovery, lying in the semi-supine position several times a day.*

Understanding the Alexander Technique

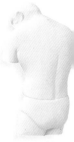

ABOVE: *Problems that have built up over many years respond to the Technique.*

THE ALEXANDER TECHNIQUE *is a process of re-education. Learning in school or at college is a process whereby a pupil gains new skills and knowledge or builds upon existing ones. In the Alexander Technique the teacher's role is more complex.*

Teaching and learning take place in the context of the person as a whole – their lifestyle, the work they do, their emotions and feelings. Added to this is the process of re-education, correcting what has been learnt inaccurately, and working toward gaining more appropriate skills. Our patterns of body movement are the result of habit – the Alexander teacher's role is to work with the pupil in recognizing habits that are unhelpful and work toward a more appropriate and balanced body use.

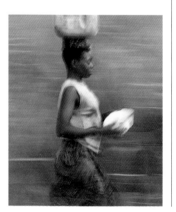

BELOW: *Natural poise and balance working well, and even being put to practical use!*

HABITS

Changing long-held habitual patterns of body use and movement is much harder than teaching something new, but this is the key to the process of Alexander Technique teaching.

Most of us approach activity and movement with little thought, and our daily movements of walking, sitting, talking, bending, lifting, reading, writing, and so on are undertaken with limited skill.

Our habits develop unconsciously, often in early childhood. We may have found life difficult and challenging, and our emotions have affected the way we hold ourselves, or we may have continuously twisted to one side when sitting and now have a spine out of alignment. The reasons we develop habits are numerous. An Alexander teacher, through observation and by using the hands sensitively, recognizes the manifestation of the habits that have developed and works with the pupil to redress the balance.

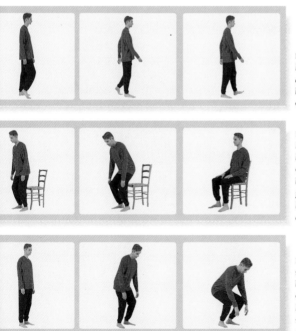

LEFT: *Utilizing the head–neck balance and maintaining length and width whilst walking.*

LEFT: *Integrating the head, neck, and back, lengthening and widening the torso, bending at the hip joint, releasing the knees, in the process of sitting.*

LEFT: *Freeing the neck, allowing the back to lengthen and widen, keeping the head–neck–back relationship intact whilst squatting.*

STOPPING TO THINK

Before we can begin to make changes in our body use, we need to become aware of what we are doing, how we are doing it, and recognize our patterns. When a pupil first works with a teacher, his level of awareness is limited, and instructions to stop or "inhibit" his response to a stimulus are difficult for him to take on board. "Inhibit" in this sense does not mean to repress, but more to stop and check what messages are being sent by the brain to the nervous system. Sometimes a teacher will have to work to bring the pupil to a state of quietness and stillness before he prevents unwanted responses. So before we make changes, we need to stop, resist responding in our habitual way, and think how we are going to do it differently.

MISLEADING FEELINGS

As we grow and develop we also acquire our own individual way of responding to stimuli. Our responses and the way in which we use our bodies, both in activity and when at rest, become comfortable and familiar. We might become aware of how we do something or how we look, but take this as a matter of course – it's just the way we are. Our habitual patterns are set and our actions feel normal.

When a teacher works with a pupil, because she has been

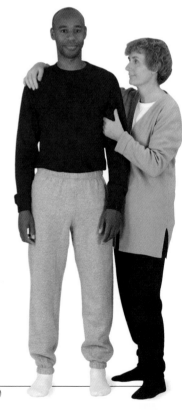

BELOW: *Alexander teachers are able to sense habitual patterns through their hands.*

30

trained to carefully observe body use, both by the visual information she is receiving and what she can sense through her hands, she will be able to see a pattern of use that is causing the body to be out of balance. The pupil's head may be tilting to one side, one shoulder may be higher than the other, or the body weight may be thrust forward.

The pupil may or may not be aware of this pattern. When the teacher brings the body weight back into balance, the pupil will feel awkward and "not quite right." Although this new state is an improvement on the established pattern, for the pupil it will feel rather strange.

The habits and patterns of use we have developed feel normal and will have taken place over a number of years – changing this to a different regime is quite a challenge. Alexander teachers are trained for three years; during this time they refine their own sensory awareness, which equips them to teach their pupils how to refine theirs. In the process, pupils usually become more generally aware of themselves as people.

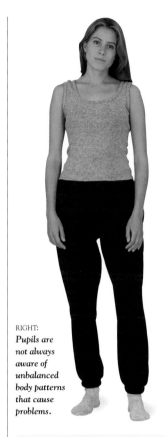

RIGHT:
Pupils are not always aware of unbalanced body patterns that cause problems.

MISLEADING FEELINGS

- Our sensory awareness of responses is unreliable.
- Habitual patterns of use feel normal to us.
- Changes in our use can initially feel awkward.

CHANGING HABITS

When we know something is wrong our natural response is to put it right. An Alexander teacher works with a pupil's kinesthetic perception, raising the pupil's awareness of the unhelpful patterns that have developed. The touch of the teacher's hands helps to remind the pupil to inhibit habitual responses and to encourage the direction that is desirable.

SARAH'S STORY

Sarah works in computers and spends a large proportion of her time on the telephone, trouble-shooting problems for customers. She is also a keen tennis player and plays two to three evenings a week, and twice at the weekend. Sarah is experiencing a stiff neck, shoulder pain, lower back pain, and pain in her knees. We have been working together for a few lessons and have identified some of the reasons for her problems.

SARAH'S PROBLEMS

Sarah has been working with her computer screen at an angle, which means she twists each time she checks the screen, and she cradles the handset between her ear and shoulder when answering queries over the telephone. When playing tennis she throws her weight forward, pulls down onto her knees, and tenses her whole body, in particular the calf and thigh muscles. Because of this, a large proportion of her weight has been focused on the knee joint, causing pain.

So far, we have worked together on changing her work situation so that the computer screen is facing her and at the right height. She now has a supportive chair at the correct height, and uses earphones and a mouthpiece for her telephone work. We are working together on her head–neck–back relationship, and the way in which she uses her whole mechanism in her approach to daily activities and tennis playing.

LEFT: *Teachers help a pupil to stop and think before going into movement.*

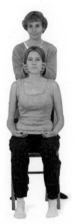

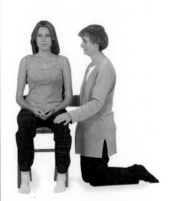

1 Sarah was taught to sit in a more poised way. At first this position felt new and strange to her.

2 Sarah was encouraged to sit without strain and tension. This was important for revising the way she worked at her computer.

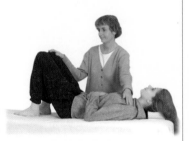

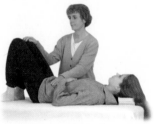

3 We worked together to undo habitual patterns of tension which Sarah had acquired over many years, and which were causing pain.

4 Sarah was shown how to release tension. This new approach helps in her everyday life, at work, and whilst playing tennis.

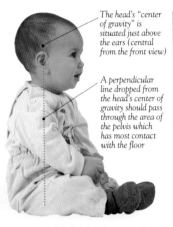

The head's "center of gravity" is situated just above the ears (central from the front view)

A perpendicular line dropped from the head's center of gravity should pass through the area of the pelvis which has most contact with the floor

ABOVE: *A baby's head is naturally balanced perfectly on the spine. Most adults lose this facility.*

THE RELATIONSHIP OF THE HEAD, NECK, AND BACK

The relationship of the head to the neck, and the head and neck to the rest of the body, is of primary importance. If this relationship is working well and in balance, it will improve the overall use and functioning of the whole of the organism. Alexander called this relationship the Primary Control, and it was the key to the way in which he worked, and is still the crux of the approach of Alexander teachers today.

The average head weighs between 8 and 12lb (4–6kg), which is quite a considerable weight to be balancing on top of the spine. Now think of this weight pulling back and down, compressing the spine, narrowing the back, and having a knock-on effect on the rest of the body. The balance of the head on the top of the spine at the atlanto-occipital joint is quite delicate, with most of the weight toward the front of the point of pivot, where the skull rests on the spine. What keeps the head in place are the sub-occipital muscles which attach the skull to the spine, shoulder blades, and collarbone.

If someone falls asleep when sitting, these muscles release and the head falls forward. When we are awake, we are unaware of the function of these muscles that keep the head in place. The average person has lost the knack of balancing the head on top of the spine with the same freedom most of us experienced when we were young children learning to crawl and walk. The majority of adults pull their heads back and down for most of the time. Whenever we go into movement or change from one position to another, the balancing process becomes even harder, and we shorten the neck muscles even more. This does not mean that a fixed position should be adopted, but rather that the balance of the head on top of the spine is ideally in a dynamic relationship.

THE RELATIONSHIP OF THE HEAD, NECK, AND BACK

- The head balance in relation to the rest of the body is of key importance.
- The balance of the head on the top of the spine is a very delicate one.
- The head/neck balance affects the co-ordination of the rest of the body.

THE SPINE

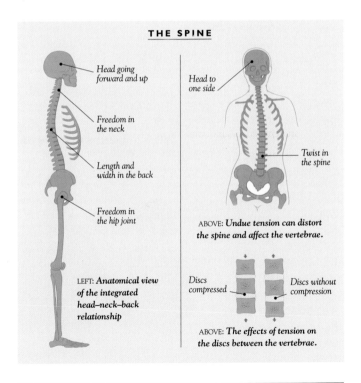

Head going forward and up

Head to one side

Freedom in the neck

Twist in the spine

Length and width in the back

Freedom in the hip joint

ABOVE: **Undue tension can distort the spine and affect the vertebrae.**

LEFT: **Anatomical view of the integrated head–neck–back relationship**

Discs compressed

Discs without compression

ABOVE: **The effects of tension on the discs between the vertebrae.**

The importance of muscles

ABOVE: *The Alexander Technique is concerned with muscle tone throughout the body.*

MOST OF US *pay little attention to our muscles, unless they ache after an activity, or we build them up for fitness, but our muscles play an important part in keeping the body in good working order. The Alexander Technique is concerned with our "use" – the way in which we consciously harness energy to approach movement.*

Our muscles play an important part in our "use," and an Alexander teacher will work with a pupil to achieve appropriate muscle tone. Muscles can have an over-active tone, when they are very tense, or poor tone, when the muscles are collapsed. Our muscle tone affects our ability to move freely, our ability to support ourselves effectively, and can affect our postural balance.

TYPES OF MUSCLE

We have two types of muscle in the body. The first, the involuntary muscles, are those that work without any conscious control from us – these include the muscles around the heart, the blood vessels, the stomach, and the intestines. The second are the voluntary, or skeletal, muscles. Most of these muscles are attached to the skeleton.

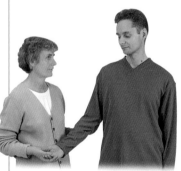

ABOVE: *An Alexander teacher shows a pupil how to release muscle tension in the arm.*

Involuntary muscles work automatically, expanding and contracting in order to keep the body working. Whatever activity we might be engaged in, or thoughts we may have, they continue to work. The skeletal muscles are referred to as "voluntary" because we have a certain amount of control over them.

MOVEMENT

Muscles have great elasticity, with the ability to contract and expand, and help us to move from one position to another. It is almost as if below our skin there is an elastic coat, and, if used appropriately, it will allow us to move with ease. However, if there is undue contraction or slackness in certain parts, everything is thrown out of balance. Often habitual contraction, developed over a period of time, actually distorts the body shape.

When we decide to move, a message is sent from the brain and transmitted through the nervous system to the muscles. So it is through our thought processes that we can change the amount of tone in our muscles. If the muscles are contracting and we think about allowing them to lengthen, we can reduce tension. Teachers work with their pupils in re-patterning the nervous system, to encourage the appropriate muscle tone to come into play.

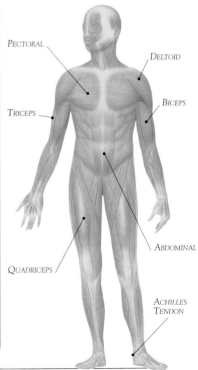

PECTORAL

DELTOID

BICEPS

TRICEPS

ABDOMINAL

QUADRICEPS

ACHILLES TENDON

RIGHT: *There are about 640 skeletal muscles. These are attached to the bones of the skeleton by ligaments and tendons.*

BREATHING

In the early days of his work, Alexander was frequently referred to as the "breathing man" because he helped people to improve their breathing. Physicians and specialists who were familiar with his work were very enthusiastic about it, and at the time this was what he was known for.

Breathing is an involuntary action, but it is amazing just how much we interfere with it. For the body to function well, there should be quiet breathing in and out through the nose, where the air is moistened, filtered, and warmed before reaching the lungs. How many of us breathe through the mouth, constantly gasp or hold our breath, or

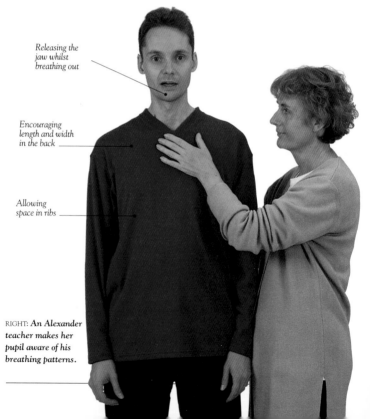

Releasing the jaw whilst breathing out

Encouraging length and width in the back

Allowing space in ribs

RIGHT: *An Alexander teacher makes her pupil aware of his breathing patterns.*

operate with rapid shallow breathing? Why is it that we enter the world being able to breathe freely and then somehow lose the knack? As with other ways in which we misuse ourselves, emotional, psychological, mental, and physical factors all play a part in interfering in our breathing.

If we tense the neck muscles, fixing the head on top of the spine, this affects the whole of the back, the ribcage, and the diaphragm. Once there is greater freedom and space in the body, less restriction in the ribcage and the lungs, our ability to breathe more freely is increased. Many people experience breathing difficulties, to a greater or lesser degree, which are often the result of tension in the upper chest and abdominal muscles.

Alexander teachers are constantly working with the pupil's breathing through the use of their hands, but they also work more specifically with the pupil on how they approach breathing. By concentrating on the out breath, pupils become aware of tensions that may be impeding their breathing.

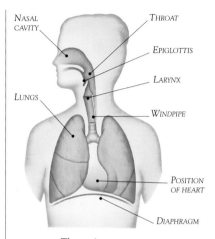

NASAL CAVITY
THROAT
EPIGLOTTIS
LARYNX
LUNGS
WINDPIPE
POSITION OF HEART
DIAPHRAGM

ABOVE: *The respiratory system. The lungs contain 600 million alveoli, where oxygen moves into the blood and carbon dioxide is passed out.*

THE KEY TO GOOD BREATHING

- Breathing is an involuntary action, and it should not be forced.
- Breathing through the nose ensures that air taken in is moistened and warmed before reaching the lungs.
- Gasping and holding the breath is linked with a tensing of the muscles.
- Our breathing is affected by the relationship between the head, neck, and back.
- Freedom and space in the body means less restriction in the ribcage and lungs.

Choosing and working with a teacher

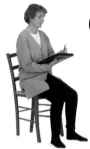

ABOVE: *At the first session, the teacher may take some notes about your case.*

PEOPLE ARE OFTEN SURPRISED *to hear that they cannot be taught the Alexander Technique in a group and that lessons need to be one-to-one. Working with the Technique is similar to learning to drive a car – you can only learn by experiencing the process on an individual basis. Introductory talks, classes, and groups have their place, but they are no substitute for individual lessons.*

Probably the most important consideration when choosing a teacher is whether or not you feel comfortable with him or her, and whether you have decided for yourself that now is the time to make some changes. Pupils who have been pressured by family or friends to take lessons may be so resistant and sceptical that the whole exercise is doomed to failure.

Your teacher will work very closely with you, gently using his or her hands to guide you. If you don't feel comfortable, choose someone else. The experiences people gain from a series of lessons vary, and depend upon why they are there and how much they want to change. How people feel at the end of a lesson differs: some people feel energized and light, and some feel heavy and want to go home and sleep. Most people experience some freedom and release, and a greater sense of well-being.

RIGHT: *Brimming with energy after a lesson!*

WHAT HAPPENS IN A LESSON?

The first lesson begins with a discussion between you and your teacher about why you have come, and about any particular problems that are of concern. Your regular daily activities will have some relevance, and these will also be discussed. Your teacher will explain the principles of the Alexander Technique and talk about some of the things you are likely to work on, and experience, during a course of lessons.

AN ALEXANDER TEACHER MIGHT ASK ABOUT...

- your general reasons for seeking lessons.
- any specific areas of concern.
- your knowledge of the Alexander Technique.
- any medical condition that could be relevant.
- any sports or hobbies you pursue regularly.

BELOW: *Learning about how the body works is a stepping stone to a better way of doing things.*

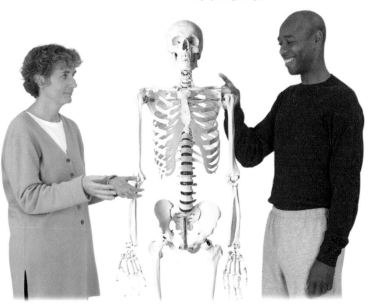

STANDING AND SITTING

Each teacher will have his or her own way of working, but every lesson involves gentle guidance with the hands and verbal instructions. These are intended to help you recognize unhelpful patterns you have developed and to teach you how to work toward integrating new patterns of use. A proportion of the lesson is spent working with the pupil in a chair, going from sitting to standing, and standing to sitting. In this way the teacher is able to highlight the head balance and work with the co-ordination of the muscles in the neck, the back, and the legs.

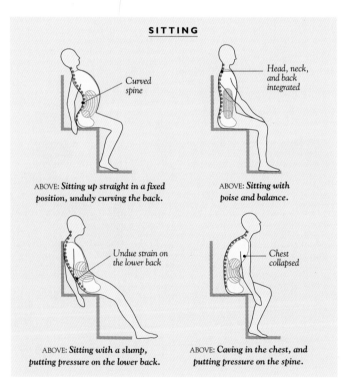

SITTING

Curved spine

Head, neck, and back integrated

ABOVE: *Sitting up straight in a fixed position, unduly curving the back.*

ABOVE: *Sitting with poise and balance.*

Undue strain on the lower back

Chest collapsed

ABOVE: *Sitting with a slump, putting pressure on the lower back.*

ABOVE: *Caving in the chest, and putting pressure on the spine.*

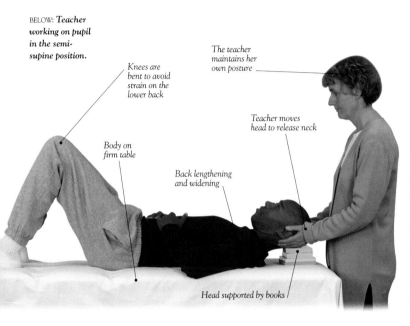

BELOW: *Teacher working on pupil in the semi-supine position.*

Knees are bent to avoid strain on the lower back

The teacher maintains her own posture

Teacher moves head to release neck

Body on firm table

Back lengthening and widening

Head supported by books

LYING DOWN

Most teachers work on a firm table, where the pupil lies down in a semi-supine position with the head supported by a small pile of books, in order to maintain the relationship between the head and neck and the rest of the body. In this position gravity has been taken out of the equation, and pupils no longer need to be concerned with supporting themselves. The teacher is able to move the arms, legs, and head, encouraging muscle release, which in turn releases the joints. Pupils are able to feel the table supporting their body and experience the release of tension as the teacher works on them.

Some pupils find this part of the teaching so relaxing that they drift off to sleep. However, they are encouraged to keep their attention fully focused and to observe the sensations they are experiencing.

EMOTIONAL
RESPONSES

The response of a pupil to the
Technique on an emotional level
will vary, some feeling very little
and others experiencing quite
dramatic changes. Some of the
emotional responses might be:

- a sense of calm and
  greater detachment.
- letting go of long-held
  habits and responses to
  people and situations.
- less dramatic mood
  swing and an ability to
  cope more effectively
  with difficult situations.
- less attachment to cravings
  such as alcohol, cigarettes,
  and certain foods.
- a greater sense of the
  connection between the
  physical and emotional state.

EMOTIONAL RELEASE

Once the basic principles of
the Technique have been
taken on board, and there is a
more dynamic relationship
between the head and neck and
the rest of the body, the pupil will
be ready to integrate this learning
into his or her daily activities.
Pupils can experience more
energy, freer movement, a greater
ability to cope with work, or a
better feeling about their bodies.

Some pupils' experience is also
on an emotional level. Releasing
long-held tensions in the body
can also release long-held
feelings – depression or anxiety
can be eased and the ability to
cope with stress enhanced. For
some, having Alexander lessons
is the first time they
have ever paid any
attention to their
body or their emotions
and feelings.

BELOW: *Some of
the emotional
benefits of the
Alexander
Technique you
may experience.*

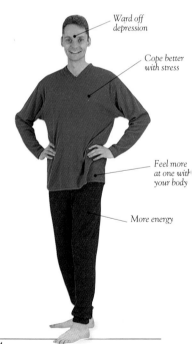

Ward off
depression

Cope better
with stress

Feel more
at one with
your body

More energy

Changing long-held habits is complex, and the help of other therapists may be required. Pupils may seek acupuncturists, homeopaths, cranial osteopaths, reflexologists, naturopaths or counsellors, or any other practitioners they feel may help.

QUALIFICATIONS

To qualify as an Alexander teacher, a candidate must complete a three-year, full-time training course. Prior to this most candidates will spend a considerable length of time working with a teacher individually, in preparation for the course. Alexander Technique students cover anatomy, physiology, the mind–body relationship, and the significance of certain medical conditions to the Technique, plus a detailed study of the books written by Frederick Alexander and other relevant authors. Training is largely practical with a very high ratio of students to teachers, and students spend a large proportion of the time working on their own body "use" with the help of teachers, before learning to work with others.

After successfully completing the course, teachers are issued with a certificate of membership from the Society of Teachers of the Alexander Technique (STAT), enabling them to use the initials MSTAT after their name. There are approximately 650 qualified Alexander Technique teachers in Britain at the current time.

IS IT SAFE?

Alexander teachers work in a very gentle way using their hands to guide the body. The amount of force that may be used is so slight that it would be unlikely to do any damage, and teachers do not manipulate the body. If, in the initial conversation about your reasons for seeking lessons, any serious medical condition is of concern, then an Alexander teacher may refer you to your physician, particularly if the latter has not already been consulted.

RIGHT: *Teachers work gently with the hands in a non-invasive way.*

Helping yourself

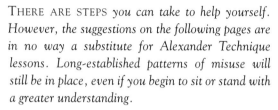

THERE ARE STEPS *you can take to help yourself.*
However, the suggestions on the following pages are
in no way a substitute for Alexander Technique
lessons. Long-established patterns of misuse will
still be in place, even if you begin to sit or stand with
a greater understanding.

ABOVE: **When**
walking freely, the
body is poised and
balanced.

The primary
movements of
the head and neck are the key to
any activity, and it is only
through experiencing freedom in
the head–neck balance that you
can begin to approach any
activity really effectively. What
the following suggestions might
do is make you more aware of
your body and how you are
using it. Observing others
can also be helpful – watch
what people do when they
are sitting, standing, or
walking. Minimizing the
amount of physical

tension we bring to any activity
helps in reducing the amount of
energy we use. If when sitting or
standing we are creating a
considerable amount of
unnecessary tension, then we
may end our day feeling tired and
on edge.

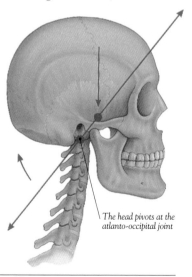

RIGHT: *Releasing tension in*
the neck at the sub-occipital
muscles allows the head to
go forward and up.

The head pivots at the
atlanto-occipital joint

SITTING

OBSERVE HOW YOU sit in a chair. Is your back supported? Are your legs wrapped around the chair legs? Are you sitting squarely or twisting to one side? Are you sitting with poise or are you slumped into the chair?

Sitting on a chair that gives support to the back, but still allows the feet to remain on the ground, is important. There are now various office chairs on the market that have been designed to give support whilst working at a desk or keyboard. For general sitting at home, a straight-backed chair is most useful. The following gives some idea of how to sit in a supported way.

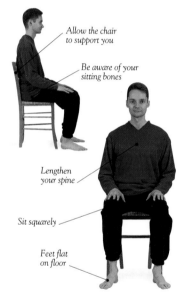

Allow the chair to support you

Be aware of your sitting bones

Lengthen your spine

Sit squarely

Feet flat on floor

1 Sit as far back in the chair as you can so that you allow the back of the chair to become a support. Think of centering your body and be aware of your sitting bones connecting with the chair. The sitting bones are the two knobbly bones at the base of the pelvis covered by the muscles in the buttocks. If you are sitting squarely on the chair, not perched, then you should feel the sitting bones.

2 Allow the weight to go down through your sitting bones, without slumping, and visualize them as a reference point from which you can then think of lengthening up the spine. Make sure your feet are flat on the ground in line with the hips.

STANDING

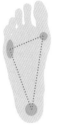

HOW DO YOU STAND? *Do you cross your arms and hunch your shoulders? Do you lock your knees at the back? Is the weight over one hip more than the other? Are you swaying back from the hips or pushing forward? Notice your feet – are the toes pointing inward or outward?*

ABOVE: **The three weight-bearing points on the foot.**

COPING WITH THE FORCE OF GRAVITY

When we stand we have to cope with the force of gravity, which takes a considerable amount of muscular effort. At the same time we have to employ the delicate skills of poise and balance using both the sensory and motor mechanisms. To do this with ease, we need to keep to a minimum the amount of muscular effort involved.

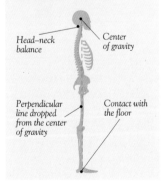

Head–neck balance

Center of gravity

Perpendicular line dropped from the center of gravity

Contact with the floor

1 *Stand with your feet about hip-width apart. Think of the weight going down the legs through to the feet and being evenly distributed. The knees should not be locked or bent.*

2 *Think of the weight going down through the ankle bone to the center of the heel. Then think of the feet as triangles, with most of the weight being distributed at the back through the heel, and then being balanced at the ball of big toe and little toe.*

3 *Allow the ground to support you and think of lengthening up the spine. The idea is neither to be fixed or slumped, but with the weight centered, so that you are not leaning forward or backward from the hip joint.*

POISED STANDING

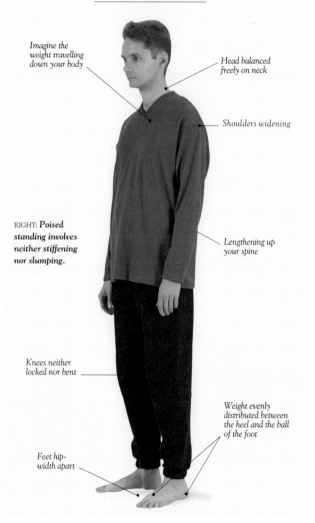

Imagine the weight travelling down your body

Head balanced freely on neck

Shoulders widening

RIGHT: **Poised standing involves neither stiffening nor slumping.**

Lengthening up your spine

Knees neither locked nor bent

Weight evenly distributed between the heel and the ball of the foot

Feet hip-width apart

LYING DOWN

IN A SERIES OF Alexander lessons you will be taught to lie in a semi-supine position, and will be encouraged to do this at least once a day for around 10–20 minutes. Lying down brings us into a state of rest where we are clearly choosing "not" to be involved in activity. It also gives the body a chance to recover and make us aware of the amount of tension we have generated. It gives the back a chance to lengthen, allows the shoulders to be released, and takes pressure off the joints.

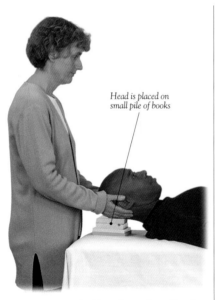

Head is placed on small pile of books

ABOVE: **An Alexander teacher will work on the head–neck relationship while the pupil is in a semi-supine position.**

1 Lie on your back on the floor – if it is not carpeted, a blanket or mat will be needed. Place a small pile of paperbacks under your head. They should be positioned under the bony part at the back of the head just above the neck, but do not allow them to press into the neck. The number of books varies from person to person, dependent upon

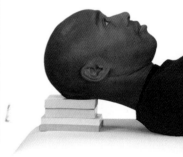

the length of the neck and the curvature in the spine.

The pile of books should be at a height where your head is not tilting backwards, and not so high that the chin is resting on the chest. Somewhere between the two will bring your head into balance and allow the neck muscles to lengthen.

2 Move your legs so that they are bent, with the feet flat and fairly near the body. Your feet should be the same width apart as your shoulders, so that the legs balance without flopping out to the sides, and are not held together too closely so causing muscle tension. The knees should be pointing toward the ceiling.

3 The palms of your hands should be resting on your stomach with the elbows resting on the floor. This position encourages greater width across the shoulders. Slide your legs down again

Be aware of lying quietly doing nothing, but focus your attention on the places where your body connects with the floor and allow the floor to support you.

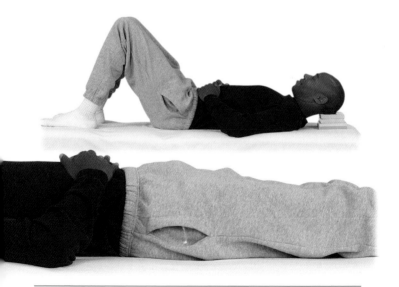

WRITING

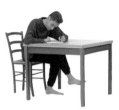

ABOVE: *Most people twist themselves into an extraordinary shape when they start to write.*

THE POSITION WE ADOPT *in order to write often goes way back to school, where we first learned to write. Are you hunched over your work? Is your head to one side? Are you clutching the pen? How much tension are you generating in your arm and wrist? Are you leaning on one elbow? Are your legs twisted around the chair?*

1 In order to write with ease the surface you use should be sloped. A manufactured writing slope is ideal, but you can create your own by using a board and supporting it underneath.

2 Make sure you are sitting squarely on your chair, with the feet on the ground, in the same way as described in the section on sitting (page 47).

3 Be aware of your wrist and allow it to be free and flexible, rather than rigid and fixed, and allow any tension in the arm to release itself.

4 Focus on how you hold your pen. Most people grip the pen tightly, which then fixes the wrist and causes tension in the arm,

and so on. Experiment with holding the pen lightly, allowing the forefinger and thumb to remain as free as possible. Try making sweeping shapes on the paper initially, and then experiment with writing. Your style of writing may change, but you will find writing in this way will take up less energy.

BELOW: *Sitting poised at a raised writing surface allows for greater freedom.*

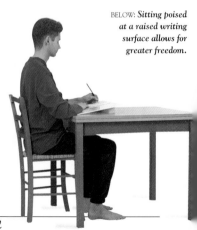

WORKING AT THE COMPUTER

TO AVOID STRAIN *on the shoulders and neck, sit at a height that allows the elbows to be level with the wrists. If the elbows drop down, the wrists will be flexed and tense. Make sure your desk and chair are at the appropriate heights. If you need to raise your chair to such an extent that your feet are not flat on the ground, use a foot rest.*

Can you view the whole of your screen easily without dropping or raising your head? Most screens on the average desk are too low and can easily be raised by using books. Sit square on, with the screen and keyboard directly in front of you. Using a copyholder is also very helpful as this helps you to avoid twisting the head to one side and constantly dropping it down to read the script and then back up to the screen.

When we sit at a screen for any length of time, it is easy to become absorbed and fixed in the way we hold ourselves. Take a break every 20–30 minutes and walk around.

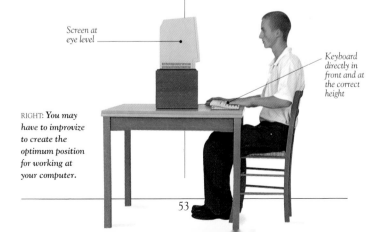

Screen at eye level

Keyboard directly in front and at the correct height

RIGHT: **You may have to improvize to create the optimum position for working at your computer.**

Common ailments

A WHOLE RANGE *of conditions are likely to improve with a series of Alexander lessons. Teachers work with the mind–body relationship and the whole of the body mechanism, not just one isolated part. The effects of lessons vary – for some people changes are dramatic, and for others there is a steady awareness that things are improving. Listed below are some of the most common conditions that have been helped by the Technique.*

HEART DISEASE

By giving the internal organs more space they can begin to operate more effectively and as tension is released, blood flow is more efficient and circulation improves. Some people suffering from heart disease find the Technique helpful in managing their condition.

HIGH BLOOD-PRESSURE

People with high blood-pressure often have the problem because they are very tense and stressed. A study carried out on music students under stress, before and after Alexander lessons, showed a significant drop in blood-pressure.

BREATHING PROBLEMS

People have breathing difficulties for a variety of

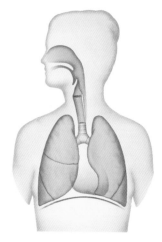

reasons, but have often developed shallow breathing, or may frequently hold their breath. In studies carried out on people before and after a series of Alexander lessons, breathing was found to be deeper, slower, and more effective afterward.

Alexander teachers will work with pupils on their general body use, which improves breathing. They will also address specific habits which may be interfering with breathing.

ASTHMA

As more space is given to the ribcage and diaphragm, lung capacity is increased and breathing improved, asthma attacks may be reduced or prevented.

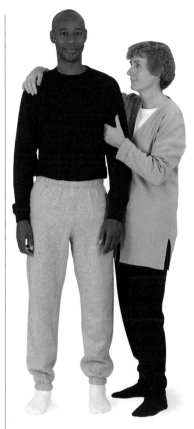

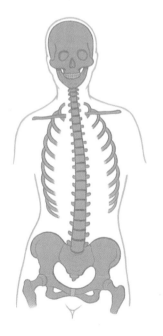

DIGESTIVE PROBLEMS

By allowing the whole body to lengthen and widen, the internal organs are given much more space in which to operate. Teachers find that various disorders of the digestive system improve with lessons.

PARKINSON'S DISEASE

A recent study of people receiving lessons showed a significant reduction in depression, a significantly more positive body concept, and significantly less difficulty in performing daily activities.

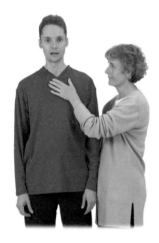

EMOTIONAL PROBLEMS

Pupils often find that as they become more aware of the mind–body connection and experience an improved sense of well-being, they begin to feel better about themselves. Many people feel invigorated and rejuvenated after lessons, which allows them to deal with emotional problems more easily.

ANXIETY

Pupils who are anxious have an opportunity to relax, work on their breathing, and learn to be in a less "excited" state.

HEADACHES AND MIGRAINE

Headaches and migraines have many causes, both emotional and physical. By working with the head–neck balance and improving general body use, pupils can reduce attacks.

STRESS

Stress is on the increase and is one of the most common causes of health problems. It can be the direct cause of conditions such as irritable bowel syndrome, chronic headaches, digestive disorders, insomnia, breathing, and skin problems. Slowing down, reducing muscular tension, and working with the mind–body relationship to improve overall responses can help those suffering from stress.

SLEEP PROBLEMS

Some pupils find that by letting go of muscular tension and improving their general body use their sleep improves, becoming deeper and more restful.

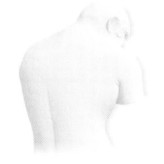

learns to reduce the pressure on the spine, the discs are given more space and allowed to regenerate, which can prevent any further deterioration.

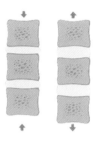

NECK PAIN

Tension in the neck muscles and an inappropriate head–neck balance will result in stiffness and pain. Once a pupil starts to work on the head–neck–back relationship, there will be a general improvement.

BACK PAIN

By improving posture, poise, and balance, reducing muscle tension, reducing the pressure on the spine, and allowing more space for the discs in between the vertebrae, back pain can be alleviated.

DISC PROBLEMS

The discs between the vertebrae are subjected to enormous pressure when there has been constant misuse of the whole of the mechanism, resulting in a variety of conditions. As a pupil

FROZEN SHOULDER

By releasing muscle tension, reducing pressure on the joints, and working with the way in which the pupil "uses" himself, frozen shoulders may be released.

ARTHRITIS

When muscular tension is reduced and posture and balance are improved, there is likely to be less strain on the joints, which can in turn help with the inflammation and pain in the joints.

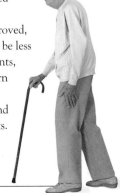

CARPAL TUNNEL SYNDROME

This is often the result of repetitive action, where the wrist has been flexed and fixed. If caught in the early stages, Alexander lessons may help to prevent this condition developing, but even those who have undergone surgery find the Technique extremely helpful.

RSI

Repetitive strain injury, or RSI, in the workplace in those using keyboards is becoming one of the fastest-growing occupational work injuries world wide. Much time and effort has been put into improving the physical environment, but little on preventing the cause. Constant inappropriate patterns of tension, combined with repetitive movement, are at the root of the problem. Once people begin to address the cause and work on the whole body use, improvements can be made.

REHABILITATION

After injury or an operation, the body is in a state of shock and people invariably experience pain. In order to cope, our natural response is to create muscular tension. Improving the whole body use can be significant in the healing and recovery process.

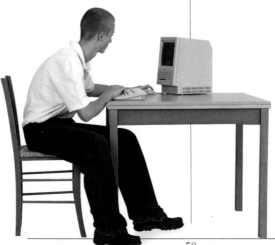

LEFT: *When working at a computer, we can develop poor habits of body use, which put us under undue stress and strain.*

Further reading

CONSTRUCTIVE CONSCIOUS
CONTROL OF THE INDIVIDUAL,
by *F.M.Alexander*
(Methuen, London, 1923)

MAN'S SUPREME INHERITANCE,
by *F.M.Alexander*
(Dutton, New York, 1910)

THE USE OF THE SELF,
by *F.M.Alexander*
(Dutton, New York, 1932)

THE ALEXANDER PRINCIPLE,
by *W.Barlow* (Gollancz, 1973)

BODY LEARNING, by *M.Gelb*
(Aurum Press, 1981)

ALEXANDER TECHNIQUE,
by *C.Stevens*
(MacDonald Optima, 1987)

THE ART OF CHANGING, by
Glen Park (Ashgrove Press, 1989)

THE ALEXANDER TECHNIQUE,
Leibowitz and Connington
(Souvenir Press, 1992)

Useful addresses

Ailsa Masterton
The North London Alexander
Practice
8C Courthope Road
London NW3 2LB
UK

**South African Society of
Teachers of the Alexander
Technique (SASTAT)**
35 Thornhill Road
Tondebosch 7700
South Africa

**The Canadian Society of Teachers
of the Alexander Technique**
PO Box 502 Station E
Montreal
Quebec
Canada 2T 3A9

**North American Society of
Teachers of the Alexander
Technique (NASTA)**
PO Box 806
Ansonia Station
NY 10023-9998
USA

**The Society of Teachers of the
Alexander Technique (STAT)**
20 London House
266 Fulham Road
London SW10 9EL
UK

**The Australian Society of Teachers
of the Alexander Technique**
PO Box 529
Milson's Point
NSW 2061 Australia